THE MEMORY BOOSTING

COOKBOOK

DELICIOUS RECIPES FOR REVERSING ALZHEIMER'S AND ENHANCING BRAIN HEALTH.

Ben S Roberts

Table of Content

introduction...7

Understanding Alzheimer's Diseases 7

The Important of Diet in Alzheimer's Reversal 9

CHAPTER 1 13

Brain Boosting Foods 13

The Best Food for Cognitive Health............................15

Recipes Featuring Brain Boosting Ingredient...............18

CHAPTER 2 21

Anti Inflammatory Foods 21

Role of Inflammation in Alzheimer's Disease...............22

Recipes Featuring Anti Inflammatory Ingredients with Prep Time and Serving Size 24

CHAPTER 3: 31

Gut Health Foods 31

The Gut-Brain Connection 32

Foods That Promote Good Gut Health for Alzheimer's patients 34

Recipes Featuring Gut-Healthy Ingredients 44

CHAPTER 4 47

Food Rich in Antioxidants...47

The Important of Antioxidant In Alzheimer's Prevention And Reversal 49

Food That Are High in Antioxidant.............................50

Recipes Featuring Antioxidants Rich Ingredients 52

CHAPTER 5 57

Low Carb, High Fat Foods 57

The Benefit of Low Carbs High Fat Diet for Alzheimer's Reversal 57

30 Foods That Are Low in Carbs and High in Healthy Fats with ingredients and prep time..............................59

Recipes Featuring Low-Carb, High-Fat Ingredients 63

CHAPTER 6 81

Meal Plan Preparation...81

Tips For Planning Alzheimers Meals 82

Tricks for Preparing Alzheimers Meal 84

Sample Of Meal Plans And Recipes For Alzheimer's Reversal 86

Day 1..86

Day 2..88

Day 3..90

Day 4..92

Day 5..93

Day 6..95

Day 7..97

Conclusion 99

The Power of Diet in Alzheimer's Reversal.................99

Final Thoughts and Recommendations 100

Understanding Alzheimer's Diseases

Alzheimer's disease is a progressive neurological disorder that affects millions of people worldwide. It is the most common cause of dementia, a term used to describe a decline in cognitive function severe enough to interfere with daily activities.

The exact cause of Alzheimer's disease is not yet fully understood, but research suggests that it is caused by a combination of genetic, lifestyle, and environmental factors. One of the hallmark characteristics of Alzheimer's disease is the accumulation of abnormal proteins in the brain, including beta-amyloid and tau proteins.

The disease typically progresses through three stages: early, middle, and late. In the early stages, a person may experience memory loss, difficulty with language, and confusion. In the middle stages, these symptoms become more severe, and a person may have trouble with basic tasks like dressing and eating. In the late stages, a person may lose the ability to communicate, and require full-time assistance with daily activities.

There is currently no cure for Alzheimer's disease, but treatments are available to help manage symptoms and slow the progression of the disease. Medications can be used to improve memory and cognitive function, while lifestyle changes like regular exercise and a healthy diet can help improve overall brain health.

Research also suggests that certain dietary patterns and food choices may play a role in Alzheimer's prevention and reversal. A diet rich in brain-healthy foods like leafy greens, fatty fish, and berries may help reduce the risk of developing Alzheimer's disease. Similarly, a low-carb, high-fat diet has been shown to improve cognitive function in people with early-stage Alzheimer's disease.

Overall, understanding Alzheimer's disease is critical in developing effective strategies for prevention and treatment. By making lifestyle changes like improving diet and exercise habits, individuals can take proactive steps to reduce their risk of developing Alzheimer's disease or manage symptoms in those already affected by the disease.

The Important of Diet in Alzheimer's Reversal

Alzheimer's disease is a degenerative neurological ailment that affects millions of individuals worldwide. It is the most common cause of dementia, a term used to describe a decline in cognitive function severe enough to interfere with daily activities.

The exact cause of Alzheimer's disease is not yet fully understood, but research suggests that it is caused by a combination of genetic, lifestyle, and environmental factors. One of the hallmark characteristics of Alzheimer's disease is the accumulation of abnormal proteins in the brain, including beta-amyloid and tau proteins.

The disease typically progresses through three stages: early, middle, and late. In the early stages, a person may experience memory loss, difficulty with language, and confusion. In the middle stages, these symptoms become more severe, and a person may have trouble with basic tasks like dressing and eating. In the late stages, a person may lose the ability to communicate, and require full-time assistance with daily activities.

There is currently no cure for Alzheimer's disease, but treatments are available to help manage symptoms and slow the progression of the disease. Medications can be used to improve memory and cognitive function, while lifestyle changes like regular exercise and a healthy diet can help improve overall brain health.

Research also suggests that certain dietary patterns and food choices may play a role in Alzheimer's prevention and reversal. A diet rich in brain-healthy foods like leafy greens, fatty fish, and berries may help reduce the risk of developing Alzheimer's disease. Similarly, a low-carb, high-fat diet has been shown to improve cognitive function in people with early-stage Alzheimer's disease.

Overall, understanding Alzheimer's disease is critical in developing effective strategies for prevention and treatment. By making lifestyle changes like improving diet and exercise habits, individuals can take proactive steps to reduce their risk of developing Alzheimer's disease or manage symptoms in those already affected by the disease.

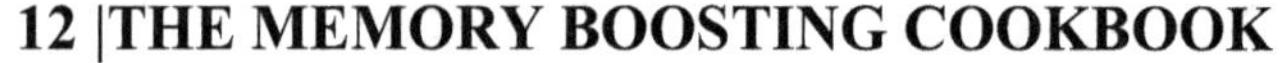

CHAPTER 1

Brain Boosting Foods

Certain foods have been shown to provide a range of nutrients and compounds that may support brain health and cognitive function. Here are some brain-boosting foods to consider incorporating into your diet:

• **Fatty Fish:** Fatty fish like salmon, mackerel, and sardines are rich in omega-3 fatty acids, which are essential for brain health. These fatty acids have been shown to improve cognitive function, reduce inflammation, and may even help prevent Alzheimer's disease.

• **Leafy Greens:** Leafy greens like spinach, kale, and collard greens are high in antioxidants and other compounds that help reduce inflammation and support brain health. They are also rich in folate, which has been shown to improve cognitive function and reduce the risk of dementia.

• **Berries:** Berries like blueberries, strawberries, and blackberries are packed with antioxidants and other compounds that help protect the brain from oxidative stress. They have also been shown to improve memory and cognitive function.

• **Nuts and Seeds:** Nuts and seeds like almonds, walnuts, and flaxseeds are rich in healthy fats, antioxidants, and other compounds that support brain health. They have been shown to improve cognitive function and may even help prevent Alzheimer's disease.

• **Whole Grains:** Whole grains like oatmeal, brown rice, and quinoa are high in fiber and other nutrients that support brain health. They have been shown to improve cognitive function and may even help reduce the risk of dementia.

• **Eggs:** Eggs are rich in choline, a nutrient that is essential for brain health. Choline has been shown to improve cognitive function and may even help prevent Alzheimer's disease.

• **Dark Chocolate:** Dark chocolate is rich in flavonoids, a type of antioxidant that has been shown to improve cognitive function and reduce the risk of dementia.

Overall, a diet rich in whole foods like fruits, vegetables, whole grains, and lean protein, as well as healthy fats and antioxidants, is key for brain health and cognitive function. By incorporating brain-boosting foods into your diet, you may be able to support optimal brain health and reduce the risk of cognitive decline and dementia.

The Best Food for Cognitive Health

Cognitive health is an important aspect of overall health, and there are certain foods that have been shown to support brain health and improve cognitive function. Here are the 10 best foods for cognitive health, along with explanations of how they may benefit the brain:

• **Blueberries:** Blueberries are high in antioxidants, which protect the brain from oxidative stress and inflammation.

Studies have shown that consuming blueberries may improve cognitive function and memory.

• **Fatty Fish:** Fatty fish like salmon, mackerel, and sardines are rich in omega-3 fatty acids, which are essential for brain health. Omega-3s have been shown to improve cognitive function and may reduce the risk of cognitive decline.

• **Leafy Greens:** Leafy greens like spinach, kale, and collard greens are high in vitamins and minerals that support brain health. They are also rich in folate, which may improve cognitive function.

• **Nuts and Seeds:** Nuts and seeds like almonds, walnuts, and flaxseeds are rich in healthy fats, fiber, and antioxidants that support brain health. They may also improve cognitive function and reduce the risk of cognitive decline.

- **Avocado:** Avocado is high in healthy fats and fiber, which support brain health. It also contains vitamin E, which has been shown to improve cognitive function.

- **Whole Grains:** Whole grains like oatmeal, brown rice, and quinoa are high in fiber and other nutrients that support brain health. They may also improve cognitive function and reduce the risk of cognitive decline.

- **Eggs:** Eggs are a good source of choline, a nutrient that is essential for brain health. Choline may improve cognitive function and may even reduce the risk of Alzheimer's disease.

- **Turmeric:** Turmeric is a spice that contains curcumin, a compound that has anti-inflammatory and antioxidant properties. Curcumin may improve cognitive function and protect the brain from damage.

- **Dark Chocolate:** Dark chocolate is rich in flavonoids, a type of antioxidant that may improve cognitive function and protect the brain from damage. It may also improve mood and reduce stress.

• **Green Tea:** Green tea contains catechins, a type of antioxidant that may improve cognitive function and protect the brain from damage. It also contains caffeine, which may improve alertness and focus.

Incorporating these foods into your diet can support brain health and improve cognitive function over time. However, it is important to remember that a healthy diet is just one aspect of maintaining cognitive health. Regular exercise, good sleep habits, and mental stimulation are also important factors in maintaining cognitive health.

Recipes Featuring Brain Boosting Ingredient

Here are some recipes featuring brain-boosting ingredients:

• **Blueberry Smoothie Bowl:** Blend frozen blueberries, bananas, almond milk, and spinach together for a nutrient-packed smoothie bowl. Top with sliced almonds, chia seeds, and fresh blueberries for added crunch and brain-boosting benefits.

• **Salmon Salad:** Mix canned salmon with chopped celery, red onion, and avocado for a brain-boosting salad. Serve on a bed of leafy greens and drizzle with olive oil and lemon juice for added flavor.

• **Spinach and Feta Omelette:** Whisk together eggs, feta cheese, and chopped spinach for a brain-boosting omelette. Serve with whole grain toast and fresh berries for a balanced breakfast.

• **Turmeric Roasted Vegetables:** Toss chopped vegetables (such as sweet potatoes, carrots, and cauliflower) with olive oil and turmeric for a brain-boosting side dish. Roast in the oven until tender and golden brown.

• **Almond Butter and Banana Toast:** Top whole grain toast with almond butter and sliced bananas for a quick and easy brain-boosting breakfast. Sprinkle with cinnamon for added flavor.

• **Quinoa and Vegetable Stir-Fry:** Cook quinoa according to package instructions and set aside. Stir-fry chopped vegetables (such as bell peppers, broccoli, and mushrooms) in olive oil and soy sauce. Serve over the quinoa for a brain-boosting and satisfying meal.

• **Walnut and Apple Salad:** Toss chopped walnuts, sliced apples, and mixed greens together for a brain-boosting salad. Drizzle with olive oil and apple cider vinegar for added flavor.

• **Green Tea Smoothie:** Blend together green tea, frozen mango, and Greek yogurt for a refreshing and brain-boosting smoothie. Add honey or stevia for sweetness, if desired.

Incorporating these recipes into your diet can help support brain health and improve cognitive function over time. It's important to remember that a healthy diet is just one aspect of maintaining cognitive health, so be sure to also engage in regular exercise, good sleep habits, and mental stimulation.

CHAPTER 2

Anti Inflammatory Foods

Anti-inflammatory foods are foods that reduce inflammation in the body. Inflammation is a natural process that helps the body heal and protect itself from disease, but chronic inflammation can lead to health problems such as diabetes, heart disease, and arthritis. Eating an anti-inflammatory diet can help reduce inflammation and reduce the risk of these and other health problems.

Examples of anti-inflammatory foods include omega-3 fatty acids, such as those found in fish, nuts, and seeds; fruits and vegetables, especially those high in antioxidants like berries and dark leafy greens; whole grains; and healthy fats, such as olive oil.

Eating an anti-inflammatory diet can also help reduce inflammation-causing foods like processed foods, refined sugars, and trans fats. Eating a balanced diet that includes a variety of anti-inflammatory foods can help reduce inflammation and improve overall health.

Role of Inflammation in Alzheimer's Disease

Inflammation plays an important role in the development and progression of Alzheimer's disease. Inflammation is a natural process that occurs when the body is fighting off an infection or injury. In Alzheimer's disease, inflammation is an abnormal response to damage in the brain.

It is believed that inflammation may cause the destruction of the nerve cells and the formation of plaque in the brain. This could lead to the symptoms of Alzheimer's disease, such as memory loss and cognitive decline. At the same time, inflammation can be a protective response to the damage in the brain.

In some cases, inflammation can actually help to slow down the progression of Alzheimer's disease. This is because inflammation can help remove the plaques from the brain and improve its function. Research suggests that inflammation is a major factor in Alzheimer's disease.

It is believed that inflammation plays a role in the development of the disease and can worsen symptoms in those who already have it. As more is learned about the role of inflammation in Alzheimer's disease, new treatments and therapies may be developed to help manage the condition.

The exact role of inflammation in Alzheimer's disease is still being studied. However, it is clear that inflammation plays an important role in the development and progression of the disease.

As more is discovered about this role, new treatments and therapies may be developed to help manage the condition.

Recipes Featuring Anti Inflammatory Ingredients with Prep Time and Serving Size

1   **Coconut Curry Lentils:** Prep Time: 10 minutes, Servings: 4

Ingredients: 2 tablespoons extra-virgin olive oil, 1 onion, diced, 2 cloves garlic, minced, 2 teaspoons curry powder, 1 teaspoon ground turmeric, 1/4 teaspoon ground cayenne pepper, 1/2 teaspoon sea salt, 1 (14-ounce) can light coconut milk, 1 cup dried lentils, 2 cups vegetable broth, 2 tablespoons freshly squeezed lime juice, 2 tablespoons chopped fresh cilantro

Instructions: Heat the olive oil in a large pot over medium heat. Add the onion and sauté until softened, about 5 minutes. Add the garlic, curry powder, turmeric, cayenne pepper, and salt, and cook for 1 minute.

Add the coconut milk, lentils, and vegetable broth, and bring to a boil. Reduce the heat to low and simmer, covered, for 15 minutes. Remove from the heat and stir in the lime juice and cilantro. Serve warm.

Baked Salmon with Turmeric-Ginger Glaze: Prep Time: 10 minutes, Servings: 4

Ingredients: 4 (6-ounce) salmon fillets, 1 teaspoon sea salt, 2 tablespoons freshly squeezed orange juice, 2 tablespoons freshly squeezed lemon juice, 2 tablespoons honey, 1 teaspoon ground

Roasted Acorn Squash with Turmeric and Cinnamon: Prep Time: 10 minutes, Servings: 4

Ingredients: 2 acorn squash, halved and seeded, 2 tablespoons coconut oil, melted, 1 teaspoon ground turmeric, 1/2 teaspoon ground cinnamon, 1/4 teaspoon sea salt.

Instructions: Preheat the oven to 400°F. Brush the cut sides of the squash with the coconut oil and sprinkle with the turmeric, cinnamon, and salt. Place the squash halves, cut side down, on a baking sheet. Roast for 30 minutes, or until the squash is tender. Serve warm.

4. Kale and Quinoa Salad with Ginger-Lime Vinaigrette: Prep Time: 15 minutes, Servings: 4

Ingredients: 1 cup uncooked quinoa, 2 cups vegetable broth, 2 bunches kale, stemmed and chopped, 2 tablespoons freshly squeezed lime juice, 2 tablespoons extra-virgin olive oil, 2 teaspoons freshly grated ginger, 1/4 teaspoon sea salt

Instructions: In a medium saucepan, combine the quinoa and vegetable broth. Bring to a boil over medium-high heat, then reduce the heat to low and simmer, covered, for 15 minutes. Meanwhile, in a large bowl, combine the kale, lime juice, olive oil, ginger, and salt. Massage the kale with your hands until it is tender. When the quinoa is done cooking, add it to the kale and toss to combine. Serve warm or at room temperature.

5. Roasted Eggplant and Garlic Dip: Prep Time: 15 minutes, Servings: 8

Ingredients: 1 large eggplant, halved and seeded, 2 tablespoons extra-virgin olive oil, 1 head garlic, peeled, 1/2 teaspoon sea salt, 1/4 teaspoon ground black pepper, 2 tablespoons freshly squeezed lemon juice, 2 tablespoons tahini, 2 tablespoons chopped fresh parsley.

Instructions: Preheat the oven to 350°F. Brush the cut sides of the eggplant with the olive oil and sprinkle with the salt and pepper. Place the eggplant, cut side down, on a baking sheet. Place the garlic cloves on the baking sheet. Roast for 30 minutes, or until the eggplant is tender.

Let cool for 10 minutes. Scoop the eggplant flesh into a food processor. Add the roasted garlic cloves, lemon juice, tahini, and parsley and puree until smooth. Serve warm or at room temperature.

6. Green Goddess Bowls: Prep Time: 15 minutes, Servings: 4

Ingredients: 4 cups cooked quinoa, 2 avocados, pitted and diced, 2 tablespoons extra-virgin olive oil, 2 tablespoons freshly squeezed lime juice, 1/2 teaspoon ground turmeric, 1/2 teaspoon sea salt, 2 cups chopped spinach, 1 cup cooked chickpeas, 1/2 cup chopped fresh cilantro

Instructions: In a large bowl, combine the quinoa, avocados, olive oil, lime juice, turmeric, and salt. Toss to combine.

Divide the quinoa mixture among four bowls. Top each with spinach, chickpeas, and cilantro. Serve immediately.

7. Turmeric-Ginger Tea: Prep Time: 5 minutes, Servings: 1

Ingredients: 1 cup water, 1 teaspoon freshly grated ginger, 1 teaspoon ground turmeric, 1 teaspoon honey (optional)
Instructions: Bring the water to a boil in a small saucepan. Add the ginger and turmeric and simmer for 3 minutes.

Strain the tea into a mug. Stir in the honey, if using. Serve warm.

8. Turmeric-Dusted Roasted Chickpeas: Prep Time: 10 minutes, Servings: 4

Ingredients: 2 (15-ounce) cans chickpeas, rinsed and drained, 2 tablespoons extra-virgin olive oil, 1 teaspoon ground turmeric, 1/2 teaspoon sea salt, 1/4 teaspoon ground black pepper.

Instructions: Preheat the oven to 400°F. Line a baking sheet with parchment paper. In a medium bowl, toss the chickpeas with the olive oil, turmeric, salt, and pepper until evenly coated. Spread the chickpeas on the prepared baking sheet. Roast for 20 minutes, stirring halfway through, until golden and crispy. Serve warm.

9.Turmeric-Coconut Rice: Prep Time: 15 minutes, Servings: 4

Ingredients: 2 tablespoons coconut oil, 1 onion, diced, 2 cloves garlic, minced, 1 teaspoon ground turmeric, 1/2 teaspoon sea salt, 1 cup uncooked basmati rice, 2 cups coconut milk

Instructions: Heat the coconut oil in a medium saucepan over medium heat. Add the onion and sauté until softened, about 5 minutes. Add the garlic, turmeric, and salt and cook for 1 minute. Stirring continuously for one minute, add the rice. As it begins to boil, add the coconut milk. For 15 minutes, or until the rice is cooked, reduce the heat to low, cover, and simmer. Serve warm.

10. Turmeric-Roasted Carrots: Prep Time: 10 minutes, Servings: 4

Ingredients: 2 pounds carrots, peeled and cut into 2-inch pieces, 2 tablespoons extra-virgin olive oil, 1 teaspoon ground turmeric, 1/2 teaspoon sea salt, 1/4 teaspoon ground black pepper

Instructions: Preheat the oven to 400°F. Line a baking sheet with parchment paper. In a large bowl, toss the carrots with the olive oil, turmeric, salt, and pepper until evenly coated. Spread the carrots on the prepared baking sheet. Roast for 25 minutes, or until tender. Serve warm.

CHAPTER 3

Gut Health Foods

Gut-Healthy Foods Gut-healthy foods are those that are rich in probiotics, fiber, and other essential nutrients and vitamins that support the health of the digestive system. These foods can help reduce inflammation, improve digestion, and protect against disease. Probiotic-rich foods are some of the most beneficial for gut health.

These include fermented foods such as kimchi, sauerkraut, miso, yogurt, and kefir. These foods contain beneficial bacteria that can help restore balance to the gut microbiome and improve digestion. Fiber-rich foods are also essential for gut health. Fiber helps to feed the beneficial bacteria in the gut and supports regular bowel movements.

Foods that are high in fiber include legumes, nuts, seeds, whole grains, and fruits and vegetables. Other gut-healthy foods include prebiotic-rich foods such as asparagus, garlic, onions, and leeks. These foods contain compounds that help to feed the beneficial bacteria in the gut. Omega-3 fatty acids, found in fatty fish and some plant-based oils, can also help to reduce inflammation in the digestive system. Finally, it is important to stay hydrated.

Drinking plenty of water will help to flush out toxins and keep the digestive system running smoothly. Additionally, it is important to reduce stress, get enough sleep, and exercise regularly to maintain a healthy gut. By following these simple steps and including gut-healthy foods in your diet, you can help to improve digestion, reduce inflammation, and protect against disease.

The Gut-Brain Connection

The gut-brain connection is a phrase used to describe the relationship between the gastrointestinal system and the nervous system. This connection is bidirectional, meaning that signals can travel from the gut to the brain, and from the brain to the gut.

The gut-brain connection is complex and involves the central nervous system, enteric nervous system, immune system, endocrine system, and the microbiome. In the gut-brain connection, the gut sends signals to the brain via the vagus nerve, hormones, and the immunity, and inflammation. The gut-brain connection is important for overall health and wellbeing.

It is believed that an imbalance in the gut microbiome can lead to mental health issues such as anxiety, depression, and other mental disorders. Research has also suggested that gut bacteria may be involved in the development of autism, attention deficit hyperactivity disorder, and other neurological disorders.

The gut-brain connection is a complex relationship, and there is still much to learn about it. However, it is clear that the gut and the brain are intimately connected and play a role in overall health and wellbeing. Taking steps to maintain a healthy gut microbiome, such as eating a balanced diet and avoiding processed foods, may be beneficial for mental health.

Additionally, lifestyle changes such as stress management and exercise, may also help to maintain a healthy gut-brain connection. In conclusion, the gut-brain connection is an important and complex relationship between the gastrointestinal system and the nervous system.

The gut sends signals to the brain via the vagus nerve, hormones, immunity, and inflammation. Research has suggested that an imbalance in the gut microbiome can lead to mental health issues. Therefore, steps should be taken to maintain a healthy gut microbiome and gut-brain connection, such as eating a balanced diet, avoiding processed foods, and implementing lifestyle changes.

Foods That Promote Good Gut Health for Alzheimer's patients

1. Yogurt
2. Kefir
3. Kimchi
4. Sauerkraut
5. Fermented Vegetables
6. Miso
7. Tempeh
8. Kombucha
9. Prebiotics
10. Probiotics
11. High-Fiber Foods
12. Berries
13. Omega-3 Fatty Acids
14. Olive Oil
15. Green Tea
16. Cruciferous Vegetables
17. Garlic
18. Onions
19. Spices
20. Apple Cider Vinegar

Yogurt Recipe:

Ingredients:

- 2 cups plain Greek yogurt
- 2 tablespoons honey
- ½ teaspoon ground cinnamon
- 1 cup fresh blueberries
- ¼ cup chopped almonds

Instructions:

1. In a medium bowl, mix together yogurt, honey, and cinnamon until blended.
2. Divide the mixture into two bowls.
3. Add the blueberries and almonds to one of the bowls and mix until blended.
4. Serve the plain yogurt in one bowl and the blueberry yogurt in the other.

Kefir Recipe:

Ingredients:

- 2 cups plain kefir
- 2 tablespoons honey
- ½ teaspoon ground cardamom
- 1 cup fresh strawberries
- ¼ cup chopped walnuts

Instructions:

1. In a medium bowl, mix together kefir, honey, and cardamom until blended.
2. Divide the mixture into two bowls.
3. Add the strawberries and walnuts to one of the bowls and mix until blended.
4. Serve the plain kefir in one bowl and the strawberry kefir in the other.

Kimchi Recipe:

Ingredients:

- 1 head napa cabbage, chopped
- 1 cup daikon radish, julienned
- 6 cloves garlic, minced
- 2 tablespoons fresh ginger, minced
- 2 tablespoons fish sauce
- 2 tablespoons gochugaru (Korean red pepper flakes)
- 2 tablespoons sugar
- 2 tablespoons white vinegar

Instructions:

1. In a large bowl, combine the cabbage, daikon, garlic, ginger, fish sauce, gochugaru, sugar and vinegar.

2. Mix until evenly blended.

3. Pack the mixture into a glass jar or airtight container and cover.

4. Let the kimchi sit at room temperature for 12–24 hours, then store in the refrigerator.

Sauerkraut Recipe:

Ingredients:

- 1 head cabbage, sliced
- 2 tablespoons sea salt
- 1 teaspoon caraway seeds

Instructions:

1. Place the cabbage in a large bowl and sprinkle with the salt and caraway seeds.

2. Massage the vegetables with your hands for 10 minutes.

3. Place the cabbage in a jar and press down firmly to pack it tightly.

4. Cover the jar with a lid and let sit for 5–7 days at room temperature.

5. Once the sauerkraut is ready, store it in the refrigerator.

Fermented Vegetables Recipe:

Ingredients:

• 2 cups of vegetables (chopped cabbage, carrots, peppers, onions, etc.)
• 2 tablespoons sea salt
• 2 tablespoons whey, sauerkraut juice, or liquid from a previous batch of fermented vegetables

Instructions:

1. Place the vegetables in a large bowl and sprinkle with the salt.

2. Massage the vegetables with your hands for 10 minutes.

3. Place the vegetables in a jar and add the whey, sauerkraut juice, or liquid from a previous batch.

4. Press down firmly to pack it tightly.

5. Cover the jar with a lid and let sit for 5–7 days at room temperature.

6. Once the vegetables are fermented and ready, store them in the refrigerator.

Miso Recipe:

Ingredients:

• 2 tablespoons white miso paste

- 2 tablespoons tahini
- 2 tablespoons apple cider vinegar
- 2 tablespoons honey
- 1 teaspoon sesame oil

Instructions:

1. In a small bowl, mix together all the ingredients until blended.

2. Store the miso sauce in an airtight container in the refrigerator.

Tempeh Recipe:

Ingredients:

- 2 tablespoons olive oil
- 1 package tempeh, cubed
- 2 cloves garlic, minced
- 2 tablespoons tamari
- 1 teaspoon sesame oil
- 2 tablespoons honey
- 1 teaspoon ground ginger

Instructions:

1. Heat the olive oil in a large skillet over medium heat.

2. Add the tempeh and garlic, and cook for 5 minutes, stirring occasionally.

3. Add the tamari, sesame oil, honey, and ginger, and cook for an additional 3 minutes.

4. Serve the tempeh over a bed of cooked brown rice, quinoa, or barley.

Kombucha Recipe:

Ingredients:

- 1 cup brewed green tea
- 1/4 cup white sugar
- 2 tablespoons kombucha starter liquid
- 1 kombucha SCOBY

Instructions:

1. Bring 4 cups of water to a boil.

2. Add the tea and sugar, and stir until the sugar is dissolved.

3. Let the mixture cool to room temperature.

4. Add the starter liquid and SCOBY to the cooled tea.

5. Transfer the mixture to a glass jar and cover with cheesecloth.

6. Let the jar sit at room temperature for 7–10 days.

7. After the desired fermentation time, transfer the kombucha to bottles and store in the refrigerator.

Prebiotics Recipe:

Ingredients:

- 2 tablespoons ground flaxseeds
- 2 tablespoons chia seeds
- 2 tablespoons hemp seeds
- 2 tablespoons psyllium husk

Instructions:

1. Combine all ingredients in a small bowl and mix until blended.

2. Store the mixture in an airtight container in the refrigerator.

3. Take 1–2 tablespoons of the prebiotic mixture per day.

Probiotics Recipe:

Ingredients:

• 2 cups plain yogurt
• 2 tablespoons honey
• 1 tablespoon lemon juice
• 1 tablespoon apple cider vinegar

Instructions:

1. In a medium bowl, mix together yogurt, honey, lemon juice, and apple cider vinegar until blended.

2. Divide the mixture into two bowls.

3. Serve the plain yogurt in one bowl and the probiotic yogurt in the other.

High-Fiber Foods Recipe:

Ingredients:

• 2 cups cooked quinoa
• 2 tablespoons olive oil
• 1 red bell pepper, diced
• 1 yellow bell pepper, diced
• 1 cup cooked black beans
• 1/2 cup sliced almonds
• 1/4 cup chopped parsley

Instructions:

1. Heat the olive oil in a large skillet over medium heat.

2. Add the bell peppers and cook for 5 minutes, stirring occasionally.

3. Add the cooked quinoa, black beans, almonds, and parsley, and cook for an additional 3 minutes.

4. Serve the quinoa mixture warm.

Recipes Featuring Gut-Healthy Ingredients

Avocado and Coconut Curry Chicken: Heat 1 tablespoon of coconut oil in a large skillet over medium heat. Add 1 diced onion and cook until softened, about 5 minutes. Add 1 tablespoon of minced garlic, 1 tablespoon of curry powder, 1 teaspoon of ground ginger, 1/2 teaspoon of dried thyme, and 1/4 teaspoon of cayenne pepper. Stir and cook for 1 minute.

Add 2 diced boneless, skinless chicken breasts and cook until cooked through, about 8 minutes. Add 1/2 cup of chicken broth, 1/2 cup of coconut milk, and 1 diced avocado. Simmer for 8-10 minutes until the sauce is thickened. Serve over warm cooked rice.

2. Kale and Quinoa Salad: In a large bowl, whisk together 1/4 cup of olive oil, 2 tablespoons of freshly squeezed lemon juice, 1/2 teaspoon of sea salt, and 1/4 teaspoon of ground black pepper. Add 2 cups of cooked quinoa, 1/2 cup of sliced almonds, 1/4 cup of dried cranberries, and 4 cups of chopped kale. Toss to combine. Serve warm or chilled.

3. Roasted Butternut Squash Soup: Preheat oven to 375°F. Cut 1 large butternut squash in half and remove the seeds. Place the squash on a baking sheet and roast for 45 minutes. Let cool.

Scoop out the flesh and add to a blender. Add 2 tablespoons of coconut oil, 1 teaspoon of ground cinnamon, and 1/2 teaspoon of sea salt. Blend until smooth. Transfer to a large pot and add 4 cups of vegetable broth. Bring to a boil, reduce heat to low, and simmer for 15 minutes. Serve with a dollop of yogurt and sprinkle with fresh herbs.

4. Baked Salmon with Ginger-Miso Glaze: Preheat oven to 375°F. Line a baking sheet with parchment paper. Place 4 (4-ounce) wild-caught salmon fillets on the prepared sheet. In a small bowl, whisk together 1 tablespoon of white miso paste, 1 tablespoon of freshly grated ginger, 1 tablespoon of honey, and 1 tablespoon of sesame oil.

Brush the glaze over the tops of the salmon. Bake for 12-15 minutes. Serve with a side of roasted vegetables.

5. Turmeric Cauliflower Rice: Heat 1 tablespoon of olive oil in a large skillet over medium heat. Add 1 head of cauliflower, chopped into small florets, and cook until lightly browned, about 8 minutes. Add 1/2 teaspoon of ground turmeric and 1/4 teaspoon of sea salt. Cook for 1 minute and then add 1/4 cup of vegetable broth. Cover and simmer for 10 minutes. Serve warm.

CHAPTER 4

Food Rich in Antioxidants

1. Acai Berries: Acai berries are a powerful source of antioxidants, containing high levels of anthocyanins, polyphenols, and other antioxidants. Acai berries are widely available in supplement form and are known for their anti-aging benefits.

2. Dark Chocolate: Dark chocolate is loaded with antioxidants, including polyphenols and flavonoids. Eating dark chocolate in moderation can help reduce oxidative stress and may even help reduce the risk of heart disease and other chronic health conditions.

3. Pecans: Pecans are an excellent source of antioxidants, containing high levels of tocopherols, phenolic acids, and other beneficial compounds. Eating pecans on a regular basis can help reduce oxidative stress, combat inflammation, and improve cardiovascular health.

4. Goji Berries: Goji berries are a superfood rich in antioxidants, including polyphenols, carotenoids, and other phytochemicals. Goji berries are widely available in dried form and can be added to a variety of dishes to boost their antioxidant content.

5. Turmeric: Turmeric is a powerful spice that is rich in antioxidants, including curcuminoids, flavonoids, and other beneficial compounds. Eating turmeric on a regular basis can help reduce oxidative stress and may even help prevent cancer.

 6. Green Tea: Green tea is a popular beverage that is packed with antioxidants, including catechins, flavonoids, and other beneficial compounds. Drinking green tea can help reduce oxidative stress, boost the immune system, and even help prevent certain types of cancer.

The Important of Antioxidant In Alzheimer's Prevention And Reversal

Antioxidants are compounds that prevent or slow down the oxidation of other molecules caused by free radicals. Free radicals are unstable molecules that can damage cells, proteins, and DNA, leading to a number of serious medical conditions, including Alzheimer's.

Antioxidants are thought to help protect against the damage caused by free radicals and may even be able to reverse some of the damage that has already been done. Studies have shown that individuals with higher antioxidant intake have a lower risk of developing Alzheimer's disease.

Antioxidants can also help reduce inflammation, which is a major contributor to the progression of the disease. In addition, antioxidants can help protect the brain from oxidative damage, which is a major factor in the development of Alzheimer's. There are several ways to increase your antioxidant intake.

Eating a diet rich in fresh fruits and vegetables is one of the best ways to get more antioxidants. Additionally, taking supplements such as vitamin C and E, as well as omega-3 fatty acids, can also help to boost antioxidant levels in the body.

In conclusion, antioxidants play an important role in the prevention and reversal of Alzheimer's disease. By increasing your antioxidant intake through diet and supplementation, you may be able to reduce your risk of developing this debilitating condition.

Food That Are High in Antioxidant

Acai Berries: Acai berries are a powerful source of antioxidants, containing high levels of anthocyanins, polyphenols, and other antioxidants. Acai berries are widely available in supplement form and are known for their anti-aging benefits.

2. Dark Chocolate: Dark chocolate is loaded with antioxidants, including polyphenols and flavonoids. Eating dark chocolate in moderation can help reduce oxidative stress and may even help reduce the risk of heart disease and other chronic health conditions.

3. Pecans: Pecans are an excellent source of antioxidants, containing high levels of tocopherols, phenolic acids, and other beneficial compounds. Eating pecans on a regular basis can help reduce oxidative stress, combat inflammation, and improve cardiovascular health.

4. Goji Berries: Goji berries are a superfood rich in antioxidants, including polyphenols, carotenoids, and other phytochemicals. Goji berries are widely available in dried form and can be added to a variety of dishes to boost their antioxidant content.

5. Turmeric: Turmeric is a powerful spice that is rich in antioxidants, including curcuminoids, flavonoids, and other beneficial compounds. Eating turmeric on a regular basis can help reduce oxidative stress and may even help prevent cancer. 6. Green Tea: Green tea is a popular beverage that is packed with antioxidants, including catechins, flavonoids, and other beneficial compounds. Drinking green tea can help reduce oxidative stress, boost the immune system, and even help prevent certain types of cancer.

Recipes Featuring Antioxidants Rich Ingredients

1. Blueberry and Spinach Salad with Honey-Lemon Vinaigrette: Start by combining baby spinach, fresh blueberries, feta cheese, and toasted almonds in a large bowl. To make the vinaigrette, whisk together olive oil, freshly squeezed lemon juice, honey, Dijon mustard, minced garlic, and salt and pepper to taste. Pour the dressing over the salad and toss to coat.

2. Roasted Acorn Squash with Pomegranate Glaze: Preheat the oven to 375 degrees F. Cut an acorn squash in half, scoop out the seeds, and brush the cut sides with olive oil. Place the squash face down on a baking sheet and roast for 30 minutes. Meanwhile, make the glaze by combining pomegranate juice, honey, and cornstarch in a small saucepan. Bring to a boil and then reduce to a simmer. Cook, stirring often, until thickened. When the squash is done, brush the pomegranate glaze over the cut sides of the squash and return to the oven for 10 minutes. Serve hot.

3. Dark Chocolate and Avocado Mousse: Place a ripe avocado, dark chocolate chips, almond milk, honey, and vanilla extract in a food processor. Blend until smooth. Taste and adjust sweetness if desired. Serve chilled.

4. Roasted Brussels Sprouts with Cranberries and Walnuts: Preheat the oven to 400 degrees F. Place Brussels sprouts on a baking sheet and toss with olive oil. Roast for 20 minutes, stirring halfway through. Meanwhile, combine dried cranberries, walnuts, and olive oil in a small bowl. When the Brussels sprouts are done, top with the cranberry-walnut mixture and return to the oven for 10 minutes. Serve hot.

5. Grilled Salmon with Mango Salsa: Start by preheating the grill to medium-high heat. Rub salmon fillets with olive oil and season with salt and pepper. Grill for about 8 minutes on each side or until cooked through. Meanwhile, make the salsa by combining diced mango, red onion, jalapeno pepper, lime juice, and cilantro in a medium bowl. Serve the salmon with the mango salsa.

6. Baked Sweet Potato Fries with Paprika-Cumin Yogurt Dip: Preheat the oven to 425 degrees F. Cut a few sweet potatoes into thin wedges and toss with olive oil and a sprinkle of salt and pepper. Spread the fries onto a baking sheet and roast for 20 minutes, flipping once halfway through. Meanwhile, make the dip by combining plain yogurt, ground cumin, smoked paprika, and a pinch of salt. Serve the fries with the dip.

7. Beet and Lentil Salad: Cook lentils according to package instructions. In a large bowl, combine cooked lentils, diced cooked beets, crumbled feta cheese, and toasted walnuts. In a small bowl, whisk together olive oil, balsamic vinegar, honey, and dijon mustard. Pour the dressing over the salad and toss to combine. Serve chilled.

8. Apricot Trail Mix: Combine dried apricots, almonds, pumpkin seeds, sunflower seeds, and dark chocolate chips in a large bowl. Serve as a snack or as a topping for yogurt or oatmeal.

9. Roasted Red Pepper and Garlic Hummus: Start by roasting two red peppers. Peel and discard the skins, then place the peppers in a food processor along with chickpeas, garlic, tahini, olive oil, and lemon juice. Blend until smooth. Taste and adjust seasoning as desired. Serve with fresh vegetables or pita chips.

10. Apple, Cranberry, and Pistachio Crumble: Preheat the oven to 375 degrees F. Combine diced apples, dried cranberries, and chopped pistachios in a medium bowl. In a separate bowl, mix together melted butter, brown sugar, flour, oats, and a pinch of salt. Sprinkle the topping over the apples and cranberries, then bake for 25 minutes or until golden brown. Serve warm.

CHAPTER 5

Low Carb, High Fat Foods

Low-Carb, High-Fat Foods Low-carb, high-fat (LCHF) foods include: -Avocado -Coconut oil -Nuts and seeds -Cheese -Eggs -Butter -Heavy cream -Olive oil -Salmon -Tuna -Chicken -Bacon -Greek yogurt -Dark chocolate -Green vegetables -Berries -Sauerkraut -Bone broth -Keto-friendly smoothies -Olives -Pork -Beef -Lamb

The Benefit of Low Carbs High Fat Diet for Alzheimer's Reversal

The Benefits of a Low-Carb, High-Fat Diet for Alzheimer's Reversal A low-carb, high-fat (LCHF) diet has been gaining popularity in recent years as a way to improve health and prevent or even reverse certain chronic illnesses. In particular, this type of diet has been studied for its potential as a treatment for Alzheimer's disease.

Studies have shown that a LCHF diet can have significant benefits for Alzheimer's patients, including improved memory, better mood, and an overall better quality of life.

The primary benefit of a LCHF diet for Alzheimer's reversal is the reduction in inflammation. Inflammation has been linked to a number of age-related diseases, including Alzheimer's. By reducing inflammation, the LCHF diet can help to slow down the progression of the disease and even potentially reverse it.

In addition to reducing inflammation, a LCHF diet can also improve insulin sensitivity and reduce insulin resistance.

This can help to reduce the risk of developing diabetes, which is a risk factor for Alzheimer's. It has also been suggested that a LCHF diet may help to reduce levels of amyloid-beta, a protein that is believed to play a role in Alzheimer's disease. Finally, a LCHF diet can provide the body with essential nutrients that can help to reduce oxidative stress and improve mitochondrial function. Mitochondrial dysfunction has been linked to Alzheimer's disease, and by improving mitochondrial function, the LCHF diet may be able to reduce the risk of developing Alzheimer's.

Overall, a LCHF diet has many potential benefits for reversing Alzheimer's disease and improving the quality of life for those living with the condition. If you are considering a LCHF diet for Alzheimer's reversal, it is important to speak to your doctor first, as this type of diet may not be suitable for everyone.

30 Foods That Are Low in Carbs and High in Healthy Fats with ingredients and prep time

1. Avocado Toast: 10 minutes, 1/2 avocado, 2 slices of whole grain bread

2. Greek Yogurt Parfait: 10 minutes, 1/2 cup Greek yogurt, 2 tablespoons chia seeds, 1/2 cup berries

3. Deviled Eggs: 15 minutes, 6 hardboiled eggs, 2 tablespoons mayonnaise, 1 teaspoon mustard

4. Cottage Cheese Plate: 10 minutes, 1/2 cup cottage cheese, 1/4 cup nuts, 1/4 cup berries

5. Kale Caesar Salad: 10 minutes, 1 cup kale, 2 tablespoons extra-virgin olive oil, 2 tablespoons Parmesan cheese

6. Baked Salmon: 20 minutes, 4 ounces salmon, 1 tablespoon butter, 1/4 teaspoon salt

7. Pork Chops with Apples: 25 minutes, 2 pork chops, 1 tablespoon olive oil, 1/2 apple, 1/4 teaspoon cinnamon

8. Baked Brie with Walnuts: 10 minutes, 2 ounces brie cheese, 2 tablespoons walnuts

9. Dark Chocolate Bark: 10 minutes, 1/2 cup dark chocolate chips, 2 tablespoons nuts

10. Coconut Curry: 25 minutes, 3/4 cup coconut milk, 1/2 cup vegetables, 1/4 teaspoon curry powder

11. Asparagus Frittata: 20 minutes, 6 eggs, 1/4 cup asparagus, 2 tablespoons olive oil

12. Avocado-Stuffed Mushrooms: 20 minutes, 8 large mushrooms, 1/2 avocado, 2 tablespoons Parmesan cheese

13. Zucchini Fritters: 20 minutes, 1 cup grated zucchini, 2 tablespoons olive oil, 1/4 teaspoon salt

14. Tuna Salad: 10 minutes, 4 ounces canned tuna, 1/4 cup mayonnaise, 1/4 cup diced celery

15. Grilled Cheese Sandwich: 10 minutes, 2 slices whole grain bread, 1 tablespoon butter, 1 ounce cheese

16. Turkey Wrap: 10 minutes, 2 slices of whole grain bread, 2 ounces turkey, 1 tablespoon mayonnaise

17. Bacon-Wrapped Asparagus: 15 minutes, 10 spears asparagus, 5 strips of bacon

18. Egg Salad: 10 minutes, 4 hardboiled eggs, 2 tablespoons mayonnaise, 1/4 teaspoon garlic powder

19. Kale Chips: 20 minutes, 1 bunch kale, 2 tablespoons olive oil, 1/4 teaspoon salt

20. Beef Jerky: 2 hours, 1 pound beef, 2 tablespoons Worcestershire sauce, 1/2 teaspoon garlic powder

21. Bacon-Wrapped Dates: 10 minutes, 10 dates, 10 strips of bacon

22. Cobb Salad: 15 minutes, 1/2 cup diced chicken, 2 tablespoons crumbled bacon, 2 tablespoons blue cheese

23. Bacon-Wrapped Shrimp: 15 minutes, 8 jumbo shrimp, 4 strips of bacon

24. Beef and Broccoli: 20 minutes, 4 ounces beef, 1/2 cup broccoli florets, 1 tablespoon olive oil

25. Tomato Basil Soup: 20 minutes, 2 cups diced tomatoes, 1 tablespoon olive oil, 1/4 cup fresh basil

26. Sweet Potato Fries: 30 minutes, 2 sweet potatoes, 2 tablespoons olive oil, 1/4 teaspoon salt

27. Grilled Cheese and Tomato Soup: 10 minutes, 2 slices of whole grain bread, 1 tablespoon butter, 1 cup tomato soup

28. Hummus and Veggies: 10 minutes, 1/2 cup hummus, 1/2 cup raw vegetables

29. Cauliflower Rice: 10 minutes, 1 cup cauliflower, 1 tablespoon olive oil

30. Chocolate Mousse: 10 minutes, 1/2 cup melted dark chocolate, 2 tablespoons almond butter, 1/4 cup coconut milk

Recipes Featuring Low-Carb, High-Fat Ingredients

1. Avocado Egg Salad

Ingredients:

2 avocados, mashed

4 hardboiled eggs, chopped

1/4 cup plain Greek yogurt

1 tablespoon Dijon mustard

1 tablespoon white vinegar

1/4 teaspoon garlic powder

1/4 teaspoon onion powder

salt and pepper to taste

Instructions:

1. In a bowl, mash the avocados.

2. Add in the chopped eggs and stir together.

3. Add in the Greek yogurt, Dijon mustard, white vinegar, garlic powder, and onion powder. Stir until everything is combined.

4. Season with salt and pepper to taste.

5. Serve immediately or refrigerate for later. Enjoy!

2. Keto Chili

Ingredients:

2 tablespoons olive oil

1 onion, chopped

2 cloves garlic, minced

1 pound ground beef

1/2 teaspoon cumin

1/2 teaspoon chili powder

1/2 teaspoon smoked paprika

1/4 teaspoon cayenne pepper

1 can (14.5 oz) diced tomatoes

1 can (14.5 oz) black beans, drained and rinsed

1/2 cup beef broth

salt and pepper to taste

Instructions:

1. Heat the olive oil in a large pot over medium heat.

2. Add the chopped onions and garlic and cook, stirring occasionally, for about 5 minutes, until the onions are softened.

3. Add in the ground beef and cook until it's browned, about 8 minutes.

4. Add in the cumin, chili powder, smoked paprika, and cayenne pepper and stir to combine.

5. Add in the diced tomatoes, black beans, and beef broth. Bring the mixture to a boil, then reduce the heat and simmer for 10 minutes.

6. Season with salt and pepper to taste.

7. Serve and enjoy!

3. Keto Fajita Bowls

Ingredients:

1 tablespoon olive oil

1 red bell pepper, sliced

1 green bell pepper, sliced

1 yellow onion, sliced

1 teaspoon chili powder

1/2 teaspoon cumin

1/2 teaspoon garlic powder

1/2 teaspoon paprika

1/4 teaspoon cayenne pepper

1/4 teaspoon salt

4 ounces cooked chicken, shredded

1/4 cup sour cream

1/4 cup shredded cheddar cheese

1/4 cup chopped cilantro

Instructions:

1. Heat the olive oil in a large skillet over medium-high heat.

2. Add the bell peppers and onion and cook, stirring occasionally, for about 10 minutes, until the vegetables are softened.

3. Add the chili powder, cumin, garlic powder, paprika, cayenne pepper, and salt. Stir to combine.

4. Add in the shredded chicken and cook for an additional 5 minutes.

5. To assemble the bowls, divide the fajita mixture among four bowls. Top each bowl with a dollop of sour cream, a sprinkle of cheddar cheese, and a sprinkle of cilantro.

6. Serve and enjoy!

4. Keto Salmon Cakes

Ingredients:

1 (14-oz) can wild-caught salmon, drained

1/4 cup almond flour

2 tablespoons mayonnaise

2 tablespoons onion, minced

2 tablespoons fresh parsley, chopped

1 egg

1/2 teaspoon garlic powder

1/4 teaspoon salt

1/4 teaspoon black pepper

2 tablespoons olive oil

Instructions:

1. In a large bowl, combine the salmon, almond flour, mayonnaise, onion, parsley, egg, garlic powder, salt, and pepper. Stir until everything is combined.

2. Form the mixture into 4 patties.

3. Heat the olive oil in a large skillet over medium-high heat.

4. Add the patties and cook for about 5 minutes on each side, until they are golden brown and cooked through.

5. Serve with your favorite sides and enjoy!

5. Keto Zucchini Pizza Boats

Ingredients:

4 medium zucchini

1 tablespoon olive oil

1/2 cup marinara sauce

1/2 cup shredded mozzarella cheese

1/4 cup grated Parmesan cheese

1/4 cup chopped fresh basil

salt and pepper to taste

Instructions:

1. Preheat the oven to 400°F.

2. Cut the zucchini in half lengthwise and scoop out the centers, leaving a ¼ inch border around the edges.

3. Brush the zucchini with olive oil and season with salt and pepper.

4. Place the zucchini on a baking sheet and bake for 10 minutes.

5. Remove from the oven and top each half with marinara sauce, mozzarella cheese, and Parmesan cheese.

6. Bake for an additional 10 minutes, until the cheese is melted and bubbly.

7. Sprinkle with chopped basil and serve. Enjoy!

6. Keto Cream Cheese Pancakes

Ingredients:

1 cup almond flour

2 tablespoons coconut flour

2 tablespoons Swerve sweetener

1 teaspoon baking powder

1/4 teaspoon salt

4 ounces cream cheese, softened

2 eggs

2 tablespoons melted butter

1/2 cup almond milk

Instructions:

1. In a large bowl, combine the almond flour, coconut flour, Swerve sweetener, baking powder, and salt.

2. Add in the cream cheese, eggs, melted butter, and almond milk. Stir until everything is combined.

3. Heat a non-stick skillet over medium heat. Grease with butter or oil.

4. Scoop 1/4 cup of batter onto the skillet and cook for about 2 minutes, until the edges are golden brown. Flip and cook for an additional 2 minutes.

5. Repeat with the remaining batter.

6. Serve with your favorite toppings and enjoy!

7. Keto Caprese Salad

Ingredients:

2 cups cherry tomatoes, halved

1/2 cup fresh basil, chopped

1/4 cup olive oil

3 cloves garlic, minced

1/4 teaspoon salt

1/4 teaspoon black pepper

1/4 cup balsamic vinegar

4 ounces fresh mozzarella, cubed

Instructions:

1. In a large bowl, combine the cherry tomatoes, basil, olive oil, garlic, salt, and pepper. Stir until everything is combined.

2. Add in the balsamic vinegar and mozzarella cubes. Stir until everything is combined.

3. Serve immediately or refrigerate for later. Enjoy!

8. Keto Chicken Parmesan

Ingredients:

1/2 cup almond flour

1/4 teaspoon garlic powder

1/4 teaspoon onion powder

1/4 teaspoon Italian seasoning

1/4 teaspoon salt

1/4 teaspoon black pepper

2 boneless, skinless chicken breasts

2 eggs

1/4 cup olive oil

1/2 cup marinara sauce

1/4 cup shredded mozzarella cheese

1/4 cup grated Parmesan cheese

1/4 cup chopped fresh basil

Instructions:

1. In a shallow dish, combine the almond flour, garlic powder, onion powder, Italian seasoning, salt, and pepper.

2. In a separate shallow dish, whisk together the eggs.

3. Dip each chicken breast in the egg mixture, then dredge in the flour mixture.

4. Heat the olive oil in a large skillet over medium-high heat.

5. Add the chicken breasts and cook for about 5 minutes on each side, until they are golden brown and cooked through.

6. Remove from the heat and top each chicken breast with marinara sauce, mozzarella cheese, and Parmesan cheese.

7. Place the skillet under the broiler for 2 minutes, until the cheese is melted and bubbly.

8. Sprinkle with chopped basil and serve. Enjoy!

9. Keto Shrimp Scampi

Ingredients:

1/4 cup olive oil

1/4 cup butter

3 cloves garlic, minced

2 pounds shrimp, peeled and deveined

1/2 teaspoon red pepper flakes

1/4 cup white wine

1/4 cup lemon juice

2 tablespoons fresh parsley, chopped

salt and pepper to taste

Instructions:

1. Heat the olive oil and butter in a large skillet over medium-high heat.

2. Add the garlic and shrimp and cook for about 5 minutes, until the shrimp are cooked through.

3. Add the red pepper flakes, white wine, lemon juice, and parsley. Stir to combine.

4. Simmer for 3-5 minutes, until the sauce is reduced.

5. Season with salt and pepper to taste.

6. Serve over your favorite keto-friendly side and enjoy!

10. Keto Coconut Shrimp

Ingredients:

1/2 cup almond flour

1/2 cup shredded coconut

1/4 teaspoon garlic powder

1/4 teaspoon salt

1/4 teaspoon black pepper

2 eggs

2 tablespoons olive oil

1 pound shrimp, peeled and deveined

Instructions:

1. In a shallow dish, combine the almond flour, coconut, garlic powder, salt, and pepper.

2. In a separate shallow dish, whisk together the eggs.

3. Dip each shrimp in the egg mixture, then dredge in the flour mixture.

4. Heat the olive oil in a large skillet over medium-high heat.

5. Add the shrimp and cook for about 5 minutes, until they are golden brown and cooked through.

6. Serve with your favorite dipping sauce and enjoy!

6. Serve with your favorite dipping sauce and enjoy!

CHAPTER 6

Meal Plan Preparation

Meal Planning and Preparation Meal planning and preparation is an essential part of any healthy lifestyle. Meal planning involves creating a plan for what meals you will make and eat throughout the week or month, while meal preparation involves actually cooking and eating them. Meal planning and preparation can help you save time, money, and energy, as well as ensure you have access to healthy, nutritious meals.

When creating your meal plan, it's important to consider your dietary needs, budget, and food preferences. Start by making a list of the meals you would like to make throughout the week or month. Consider what ingredients you will need to purchase, and make sure to make a shopping list before you go to the store.

Once you've made your meal plan, it's time to start prepping and cooking. Start by prepping any ingredients that require advance preparation, such as chopping vegetables, marinating meats, or soaking beans. Then, cook the meals you've planned for the week. If you're short on time, you can also cook some meals ahead of time and store them for later use.

Finally, make sure to store any leftovers in airtight containers and store them in the refrigerator or freezer so you can enjoy them for future meals. Meal planning and preparation is a great way to make sure you have access to healthy, nutritious meals throughout the week.

Tips For Planning Alzheimers Meals

1 Choose nutrient-dense ingredients: Focus on adding nutrient-dense ingredients to your meals. This means including fresh fruits and vegetables, lean proteins, whole grains, healthy fats, and foods with omega-3 fatty acids and other antioxidants.

2. Avoid processed foods: Processed foods can be high in sugar, unhealthy fats, and sodium and can contribute to inflammation. Instead, opt for fresh, whole foods that are cooked at home.

3. Make portion sizes appropriate: Portion sizes can play an important role in managing blood sugar levels, so be sure to plan meals that are appropriate for the person's caloric needs. 4. Add herbs and spices: Herbs and spices can add flavor to meals and can also provide additional antioxidant and anti-inflammatory benefits.

5. Include healthy fats: Healthy fats are important for brain health and can help to reduce inflammation. Be sure to include healthy fats like olive oil and nuts in your meals.

6. Include probiotics: Probiotics can help to maintain a healthy gut, which is important for overall health. Look for probiotic-rich foods like Greek yogurt, kimchi, and sauerkraut.

7. Limit added sugars: Added sugars can contribute to inflammation and can lead to blood sugar spikes. Be sure to limit added sugars in your meals. 8. Stay hydrated: Staying hydrated is important for overall health and can help to manage inflammation. Be sure to include plenty of water in your meals.

Tricks for Preparing Alzheimers Meal

1. Stick to a Nutrient-Rich Diet: A healthy diet for Alzheimer's reversal should include plenty of fruits, vegetables, whole grains, lean proteins, and healthy fats. Avoid processed foods, fried foods, and sugary foods.

2. Use Healthy Fats: Healthy fats are essential for brain health and can help reduce inflammation that can lead to Alzheimer's. Use olive oil, nuts, seeds, and avocados in your meals.

3. Get Plenty of Vitamins: Vitamins A, B, C, D, and E are all essential for proper brain function. Make sure to get plenty of these vitamins through food or supplements.

4. Incorporate Herbs and Spices: Adding herbs and spices to your meals can help improve cognitive function and reduce inflammation. Turmeric, rosemary, sage, and ginger are all good choices.

5. Make Brain-Boosting Smoothies: Smoothies are a great way to get a lot of nutrition in one quick and easy meal. Try blending fruits, vegetables, nuts, seeds, and healthy fats for a delicious and nutritious smoothie.

6. Choose Low-Glycemic Foods: High-glycemic foods, such as white bread and refined sugars, can cause spikes in blood sugar that can damage brain cells. Choose low-glycemic foods, such as whole grains and complex carbohydrates, for better brain health.

7. Drink Green Tea: Green tea is rich in antioxidants that can help protect the brain and reduce inflammation. Try drinking a cup of green tea every day for improved brain health.

8. Eat Fish: Fish is packed with omega-3 fatty acids, which are essential for brain health. Try to eat a few servings of fish each week for the best results.

9. Get Enough Sleep: Sleep is essential for proper brain function. Make sure to get at least eight hours of sleep each night for maximum brain health.

10. Use Probiotics: Probiotics are beneficial bacteria that can help improve digestion and reduce inflammation. Try adding probiotics to your diet to help improve your brain health.

Sample Of Meal Plans And Recipes For Alzheimer's Reversal

Day 1

Meal Plan:

Breakfast: Kale, Spinach, and Tomato Omelet

Lunch: Grilled Salmon with Roasted Asparagus

Dinner: Cauliflower and Zucchini Lasagna

Recipe:

Kale, Spinach, and Tomato Omelet

Ingredients:

• 2 tablespoons olive oil

• 1/4 cup diced onion

• 2 cups chopped kale

• 2 cups baby spinach

• 1/2 cup diced tomatoes

• 4 eggs

• 2 tablespoons shredded cheese

• Salt and pepper to taste

Instructions:

1. In a big skillet, warm the olive oil over medium heat.

2. Include the onion and simmer for a further 2 to 3 minutes, or until soft.

3. Add the kale, spinach, and tomatoes and cook for 5 minutes, or until the vegetables are tender.

4. Beat the eggs and season them with salt and pepper in a different bowl.

5. Pour the egg mixture into the skillet and cook until the eggs are set, about 5 minutes.

6. Sprinkle with cheese and cook for an additional minute.

7. Serve warm.

Day 2

Meal Plan:

Breakfast: Avocado Toast with Egg

Lunch: Quinoa Salad with Roasted Vegetables

Dinner: Baked Cod with Roasted Sweet Potatoes

Recipe:

Avocado Toast with Egg

Ingredients:

• 2 slices whole grain bread

• 1 avocado, mashed

• 2 eggs

• Salt and pepper to taste

Instructions:

1. Toast the bread until golden brown.

2. Spread the mashed avocado onto the toast.

3. Heat a nonstick skillet over medium heat and add the eggs.

4. Cook the eggs until the whites are set and the yolks are still runny, about 3 minutes.

5. Place the eggs on top of the avocado toast.

6. Sprinkle with salt and pepper.

7. Serve warm.

Day 3

Meal Plan:

Breakfast: Overnight Oats with Berry Compote

Lunch: Lentil Soup

Dinner: Baked Turkey Breast with Roasted Root Vegetables

Recipe:

Overnight Oats with Berry Compote

Ingredients:

- 1 cup rolled oats

- 1 cup almond milk

- 1/4 cup chia seeds

- 1 teaspoon ground cinnamon

- 1/4 cup mixed berries

- 2 tablespoons honey

- 1 teaspoon lemon juice

Instructions:

1. In a bowl, combine the oats, almond milk, chia seeds, and cinnamon.

2. Mix until well combined and transfer to a mason jar or other airtight container.

3. Refrigerate overnight.

4. In a small saucepan, combine the berries, honey, and lemon juice.

5. Bring to a boil, reduce heat, and simmer for 10 minutes or until the compote is thick and syrupy.

6. Serve the oats topped with the berry compote.

Day 4

Meal Plan:

Breakfast: Blueberry Smoothie

Lunch: Salmon Burgers with Avocado

Dinner: Roasted Vegetable and Quinoa Bowl

Recipe:

Blueberry Smoothie

Ingredients:

- 1 cup frozen blueberries

- 1 banana

- 1/2 cup almond milk

- 1 tablespoon chia seeds

- 1 tablespoon honey

- 1/2 teaspoon ground cinnamon

Instructions:

1. Place all ingredients in a blender and blend until smooth.

2. Serve immediately.

Day 5

Meal Plan:

Breakfast Scrambled Eggs with Spinach and Mushrooms

Lunch: : Quinoa and Black Bean Salad

Dinner: Baked Chicken with Roasted Broccoli

Recipe:

Scrambled Eggs with Spinach and Mushrooms

Ingredients:

• 2 tablespoons olive oil

• 1 cup sliced mushrooms

• 1/2 cup chopped spinach

• 4 eggs

• 2 tablespoons shredded cheese

• Salt and pepper to taste

Instructions:

1. Heat the olive oil in a large skillet over medium heat.

2. Add the mushrooms and cook for 3-4 minutes, or until softened.

3. Add the spinach and cook for an additional minute.

4. In a separate bowl, beat the eggs and season with salt and pepper.

5. Pour the egg mixture into the skillet and cook until the eggs are set, about 5 minutes.

6. Sprinkle with cheese and cook for an additional minute.

7. Serve warm.

Day 6

Meal Plan:

Breakfast: Oatmeal with Apples and Walnuts

Lunch: Lentil and Vegetable Soup

Dinner: Baked Salmon with Roasted Brussels Sprouts

Recipe:

Oatmeal with Apples and Walnuts

Ingredients:

• 1 cup rolled oats

• 2 cups water

• 1 apple, cored and diced

• 1/4 cup chopped walnuts

• 1 teaspoon ground cinnamon

• 2 tablespoons honey

Instructions:

1. Heat the water to a rolling boil in a medium saucepan.

2. Stir in the oats, then lower the heat to low.

3. Simmer for 5 minutes or until the oats are cooked.

4. Add the diced apple, walnuts, cinnamon, and honey.

5. Cook for an additional 2 minutes or until the apples are tender.

6. Serve warm.

Day 7

Meal Plan:

Breakfast: Banana and Almond Butter Toast

Lunch: Grilled Veggie Sandwich

Dinner: Baked Tofu with Roasted Potatoes

Recipe:

Banana and Almond Butter Toast

Ingredients:

• 2 slices whole grain bread

• 2 tablespoons almond butter

• 1 banana, sliced

• 1 tablespoon honey

Instructions:

1. Toast the bread until golden brown.

2. Spread the almond butter onto the toast.

3. Top with the banana slices and drizzle with honey.

4. Serve warm.

The Power of Diet in Alzheimer's Reversal

The power of diet in Alzheimer's reversal cannot be overstated. The recipes and dietary guidelines provided in this cookbook have been carefully curated to help people with Alzheimer's disease and their loved ones maintain a healthy diet that can improve brain function and overall health. By incorporating nutrient-dense foods, healthy fats, and limiting processed foods and sugars, individuals with Alzheimer's can experience improvements in cognitive function, memory, and even behavior. It is important to remember that a healthy diet is just one aspect of managing Alzheimer's disease, and it should always be combined with appropriate medical care and other lifestyle modifications. Nonetheless, this cookbook provides a valuable resource for those seeking to incorporate healthy dietary habits into their lives and potentially reverse the effects of Alzheimer's disease.

Final Thoughts and Recommendations

In conclusion, the Alzheimer's cookbook provides an excellent resource for individuals and families seeking to incorporate healthy dietary habits into their lives. The recipes and dietary guidelines presented in this cookbook are based on sound scientific research and have been carefully curated to provide the necessary nutrients and dietary components to improve brain function and overall health in individuals with Alzheimer's disease.

Furthermore, the cookbook is user-friendly and easy to follow, making it accessible to a wide range of readers. The inclusion of practical tips and nutritional information also adds to its value, helping readers make informed decisions about their diets and food choices.

I highly recommend the Alzheimer's cookbook to individuals and families who are looking to manage Alzheimer's disease through diet and lifestyle changes.

However, it is important to remember that a healthy diet is just one aspect of managing Alzheimer's disease and that medical care and other lifestyle modifications are also important. Therefore, I suggest consulting with a healthcare professional before making any significant dietary changes or beginning a new exercise routine. Overall, the Alzheimer's cookbook is an excellent resource for anyone looking to improve their brain function and overall health through dietary changes.